Hiking NJ Trails

Hunterdon County & Beyond

You Can Get There From Here Too

ALICE OLDFORD

CONTENTS

ACKNOWLEDGMENTS

Special thanks to Jim Graham, intrepid walking partner/friend, photographer for our adventures and explorations on the trails in all seasons.

Thanks to Judy Loose for her technical expertise working with my cover design, formatting and website.

Kudos to Laura Gooley-Trout and Matthew Gooley who took to the trails to capture some additional photos.

Mike Helbing, extreme hiker and co-founder of Metrotrails, got us on track in our quest to explore the Highlands Trail. His dedication to hiking and trail development helps keep hiking in NJ a reality.

Heartfelt thanks to my husband, friends and Sunrise Circle Writers for their continued support and encouragement.

INTRODUCTION
WHERE WE'VE BEEN

Chances are you've read *You Can Get There from Here: Hiking Hunterdon County Trails.* You will find it a good companion for this book. Taking a friend or family along on outings adds to the fun and safety. My willing companion/photographer is Jim Graham.

If you're as avid about getting out there as we are, you may be looking to broaden your base a bit. Hunterdon, Warren and Morris Counties are all part of the Skylands Region of northwest New Jersey. Ridges, valleys and country roads invite everyone with walking shoes outside to enjoy the best that nature has to offer.

As in the first book our degree of difficulty descriptions are subjective "easy" being suitable for folks with good sneakers who spend more time in the work environment than exercising. Easy works, too, for families with children approximately 8 years of age and under. Sore muscles on your return to work on Monday should not be an issue.

Moderate suggests sturdier shoes and certainly a water bottle. If you are bringing the family, we believe children 9 to 12 could appreciate these trails. There is likely to be some rolling terrain. Moderate could cause you to break a sweat and be aware of your muscles that have spent a sedentary week. If you do get in some walking or time in the gym during the week, moderate will be fun.

Let's say you need a challenge, either for body or mind, go for difficult. Be sure you have hiking shoes, water and perhaps a snack. You will encounter rocks, even boulders, and some steep hills. Children ages 13 and up should be able to handle these trails.

By all means, bring your camera. Seasonally there are all sorts of things of interest you might want to share from gnomes in spring (I believe they travel south in winter) to glistening virgin snow in winter.

WHAT'S NEW?
Highlands Trail

If you've been hiking in Hunterdon and exploring the trails, you are aware of the Highlands Trail, a self-described "rugged footpath," extending from Storm King Mountain on the Hudson River in NY south to Riegelsville, NJ on the Delaware River. This is a volunteer project of the New York New Jersey Trail Conference. Please do check out their website at www.highlands-trail.org.

You may have tried to find the connections in Hunterdon and been frustrated in that quest. We've met one of the developers and founder of Metrotrails, extreme hiker Mike Helbing, who gave us some valuable insights.

Some of the segments in Hunterdon lend to day hikes. The beginning point is to know what you're looking for and then make a plan. First, be aware that you are seeking teal diamond blazes, and two blazes together indicate a turn. You may also see some white diamonds declaring the trail to be part of the Highlands Trail.

The Highlands Trail typically does not have the "amenities," if you will, offered by the County or State Parks trails – no restroom facilities or parking. The trail tends to take you through the woods and connect via roads.

The Highlands Trail sections do highlight the beauty of the Highlands region. Eventually, the 150-mile route will connect major scenic attractions in NJ and NY.

These trails probably do not lend to family hiking, and to our way of thinking are best undertaken in the fall or early spring. Hiking shoes and long pants are in order.

Metrotrails.org

Fifteen years in development, Metrotrails was officially established as a NJ non-profit organization in 2010. Its stated mission: *The purpose of Metrotrails is to assist in the planning, development, maintenance, and promotion of trail systems in the New York/Philadelphia metropolitan area, as well as education and preservation of natural and historic aspects of their routes.*

Metrotrails grew from a hiking group Mike Helbing initiated in 1997 in honor of his 17th birthday. The group meets consistently each weekend hiking 15-20 miles throughout the region. Mike has led more than 651 hikes, and annually the group can count on hiking the Warren Railroad in recognition of its beginning. Check out Mike's book, *Hiking the Warren Railroad Mile-by-Mile.* For more information contact Mike at sneezehorse@hotmail.com.

Now you're ready to go. Remember long pants and sturdy shoes together with a water bottle are must have equipment. A daypack with bug spray, tissues, energy bar, rain gear, perhaps a flashlight, this book and maps put you on track for a great outdoor experience.

Alice Oldford

HUNTERDON COUNTY

CHAPTER 1
CUSHETUNK MOUNTAIN NATURE PRESERVE CONNECTOR

If you can find a path with no obstacles, it probably doesn't lead anywhere.

Difficulty: Moderate to Challenging
Distance: 2-4 miles
Location: Clinton and Readington Townships
Sun/shade: Mostly shade
Highlights: Views, rocks, solitude
Restrooms: No
Parking: Dirt and gravel
Hunting: Yes
Directions:

> From Clinton, take Route 22 east. Turn right at Rt. 629, also known as the Round Valley Access Road. Proceed 1.4 miles and turn left at the Boat Launch Ramp. Follow this road for another 1.4 miles to Old Mountain Road. Turn right and travel 1.5 miles. Parking for the park is just before the railroad tracks on the right.

The mountains, adjacent to Round Valley Reservoir, were formed by volcanic activity over 160 million years ago. The Lenni Lenape Indians called the area Cushetunk, which means place of hogs; and you can almost envision the wild hogs traversing the narrow trails.

As a result of the steep inclines, the Cushetunk Mountain trail connector to Pickell Park is definitely not for the faint of heart. Long pants are in order together with bug spray and hiking shoes. Do not forget your water, and chances are you would be glad for an energy bar. I always think of this trail as ideally suited to contemplation or meditation.

Certainly it is a great place for an attitude adjustment as needed.

If you are taking kids along, I would think 8 - 10 and up could enjoy the hike.

We started out from the parking lot along the Scout Trail with yellow blazes, determined to make our way to Pickell Park in Readington Township. It was summer and lovely to be in the shade. The Scout Trail connects with the Connector Trail marked with blue blazes. We found although the Connector Trail gains almost as much elevation as the Ridge Trail, the switchbacks make it more gradual than the Ridge Trail, which is pretty much straight up. At the point where we needed to make a decision to follow the actual connector, we were drawn to the Ridge Trail hoping for some views. The Ridge Trail is closed April 1 to August 1 so as not to disturb the nesting eagles.

Although the views proved elusive because of the leaves, there was a nice cool breeze along the ridge. This very rocky trail is well marked with white markers if a little overgrown due to lack of use since it was early in August.

What a great 2.5 mile serious walk in the woods. Because of the rocks, the going is slow, and it took us nearly 3 hours to make the loop.

It occurred to us that rather than simply out and back on the connector, two cars might be in order for the 4 mile sojourn from parking lot to parking lot.

Exploration of the Pickell Park end of the Connector Trail will be an adventure for another day.

To control the deer population, hunting is allowed in the Park with a special hunting license issued by the County Park System in addition to the NJ Division of Fish and Wildlife license. There are 380 huntable acres, and 20 permits are issued.

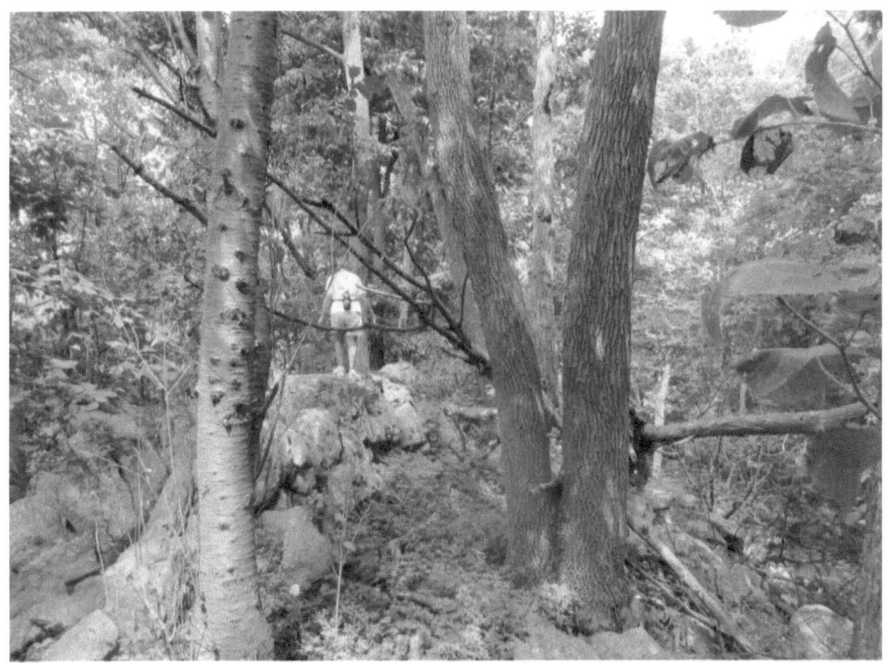

Jim Graham

Alice Oldford

CHAPTER 2
PICKELL PARK

Energy and persistence conquer all things.
Benjamin Franklin

Difficulty: Easy to challenging
Distance: 1-4 miles
Location: Readington to Clinton Township
Sun/shade: Shade and sun
Highlights: Farm fields, mountains, views
Restrooms: Yes
Parking: Paved
Hunting: No in Readington, Yes in County Park
Directions:

> From Clinton, take Route 22 east. Turn right at Rt.
> 523, then right on Mountain Road. Parking is behind
> the Municipal building.

The park offers something for everyone, including softball/t-ball fields, tennis courts, basketball court and playground. Additionally, there is a gazebo/picnic area. If walking is your goal, easily accessed from the parking lot, there are some very easy loop trails, which be forewarned could be wet, around the former Vislocky Farm. Or, you may be drawn to the Cushetunk mountain trails and views of Round Valley Reservoir.

Long pants are in order together with bug spray and hiking shoes. The blue-blazed trail connects with the Hunterdon County Cushetunk Mountain Preserve.

Once you start up the mountain the hiking gets serious. There are lots of rocks and rough going, which probably make this unsuitable for young children. You can follow the Connector Trail all the way from Pickell Park to the Old Mountain Road parking area for the County Cushetunk Mountain Preserve.

Or there are options to choose to access the summit and views of Round Valley assuming foliage does not impede the views. Check out a scenic alternative called the "Old Dam Loop," which passes stone remains of an old water impoundment.

Remember, once you get into the Cushetunk Mountain Preserve, the Ridge Trail is closed April 1 to August 1 so as not to disturb the nesting eagles.

Please do read the chapter on the Cushetunk Mountain connector trail for details.

We really recommend a car at each end, one car at Pickell Park and one car at the Old Mountain Road parking for Cushetunk Mountain Preserve, to maximize your enjoyment of this hike.

To control the deer population, hunting is allowed in the Hunterdon County Park with a special hunting license issued by the County Park System in addition to the NJ Division of Fish and Wildlife license. There are 380 huntable acres in Cushetunk Mountain Preserve, and 20 permits are issued.

CHAPTER 3
HIGHLANDS CONNECTOR FROM THE COLUMBIA TRAIL

Motivation is what gets you started.
Habit is what keeps you going.
Jim Ryun

Difficulty: Easy to Moderate
Distance: 4 miles +
Location: High Bridge Borough, Clinton and Lebanon Townships
Sun/shade: Mostly shade
Highlights: Views, gorge, dam
Restrooms: No
Parking: Gravel
Hunting: No
Directions:

> To Parking in High Bridge. From Rt. 31 go north on Route 513. Follow Rte. 513 into High Bridge. After about 1 mile and passing under the trail tracks, turn left into the center of High Bridge. Follow signs to the High Bridge Commons parking area on the left.

You already know about the Columbia Trail, the most

popular trail in Hunterdon County, but did you know there is a Highlands Connector trail that you can pick up?

Take the Columbia Trail from High Bridge to the 2 ½ mile marker or from Califon to the 4 ½ mile marker. You will see the teal blazes that are the guides for Highlands Trail. It is a single track, switchback trail up the hill. In the fall there are views of the Ken Lockwood Gorge. Do keep the trail markers in view. Eventually you come to what appears to be part of a driveway. Yes, that is part of the trail. There is also a small abandoned cabin which is kind of fun to explore.

You come out to Rt. 513 near the intersection of Bunnvale Road and the Bunnvale Library. Now you have some choices. You can proceed south on Rt. 513 to Voorhees Park where you can continue your sojourn on the Highlands Trail; or if you've had enough fun for one day, you might have chosen to leave a second car at the Library.

Consider long pants, bug spray and sturdy shoes. This is a nice outing, not too difficult, for mid-size kids say 6 – 10 years.

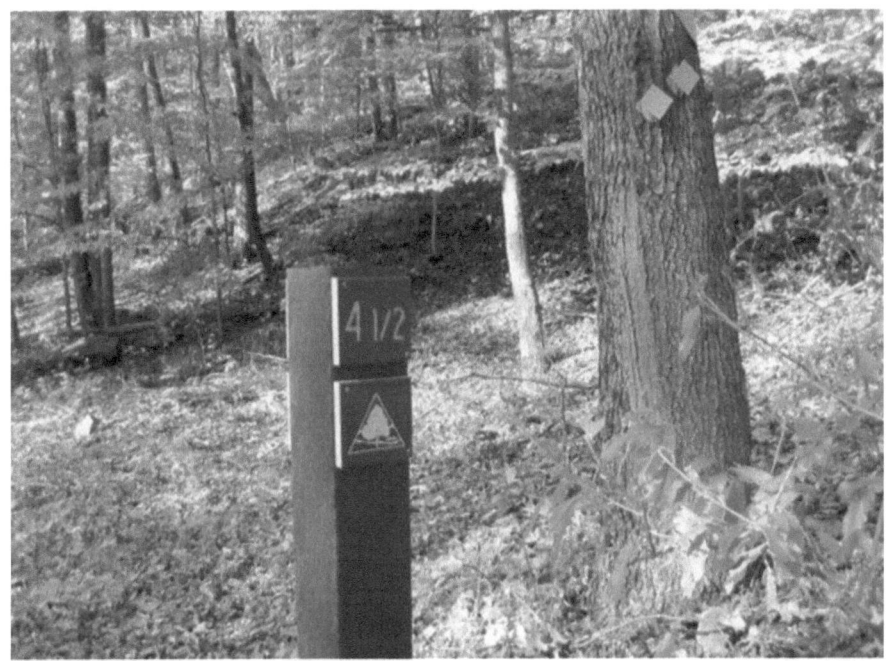

Jim Graham

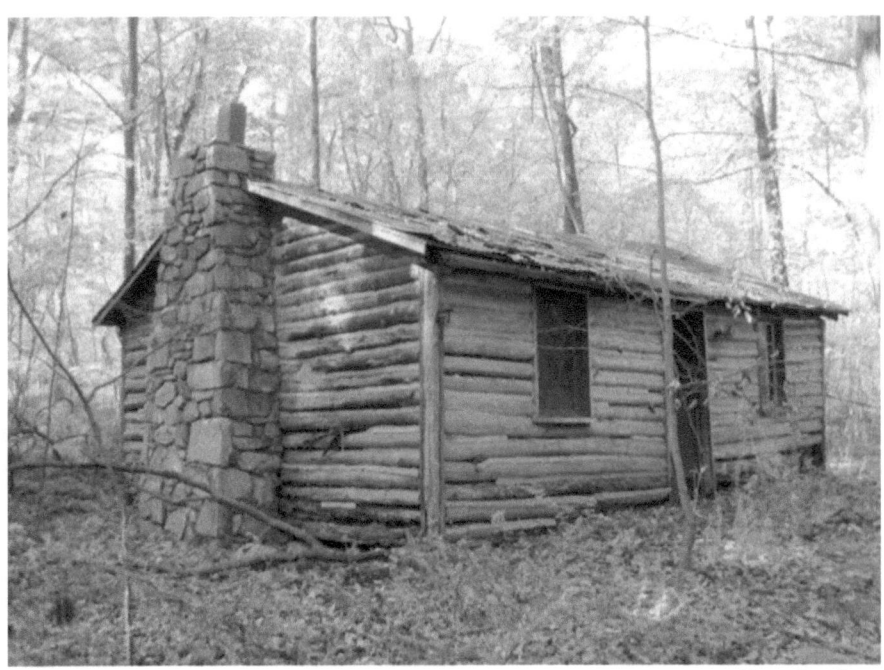

Jim Graham

Alice Oldford

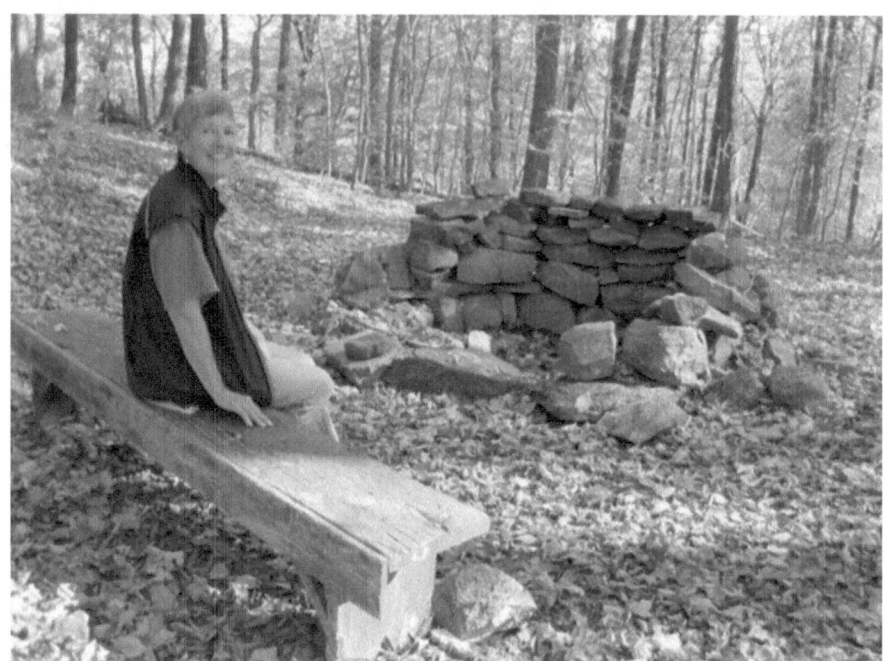

Jim Graham

CHAPTER 4
TAYLOR STEELWORKERS HISTORIC GREENWAY

Do just once what others say you can't do, and you will never pay attention to their limitations again.
James R. Cook

Difficulty: Moderate to Challenging
Distance: 6.2 miles
Sun/Shade: Mostly shady
Location: High Bridge
Highlights: Historic buildings, Solitude falls, Lake Solitude, wildlife viewing
Restrooms: Portajohn at parking area
Parking: Gravel at High Bridge Commons
Hunting: No
Fishing: Yes
Directions:
> Rt. 513N into High Bridge. Park in High Bridge Commons lot.

This trail was conceived by the Union Forge Heritage Association to honor the legacy of the working men and women of the Taylor Wharton Iron and Steel Company (TISCO). Founded in 1742, the Union Forge Iron Works is the oldest foundry in the history of the United States. Solitude Falls produced the hydroelectric power to run the operations. The stone TISCO office building, a state and nationally recognized historic structure, dates to 1725. It has been placed on Preservation New Jersey's top 10 list of endangered site.

Solitude House built in 1712 pre-dates High Bridge itself. George and Martha Washington visited the house during the Revolutionary period, and John Penn, the last royal governor of Pennsylvania was imprisoned at Solitude House for 7 months during the Revolutionary War. In 2002 Union Forge Heritage Association opened the Solitude House as a museum. Unfortunately, at this writing in September 2012, High Bridge has not extended the lease, and the museum will be closed till further notice.

The final stop on the trail is Springside Farm, which was the center of agricultural and dairy operations for the complex.

Union Forge Heritage Association has detailed the history of the historic structures on 6 trail markers.

We encourage you to take your time to appreciate the rich history made accessible through the efforts of Union Forge Heritage Association.

All that said, let's get started. This is a wonderful mostly shady walk for a hot summer's outing. Park in the High Bridge Commons lot and walk out the Columbia Trail approximately ¼ mile from its starting point. You cannot miss the large County sponsored sign designating the start of the Taylor Steelworkers Historic Greenway trail. The trail is single track in many places with lots of vegetation, so we strongly recommend long pants and sturdy shoes. Once you start down the trail, plan to take in the view of Lake Solitude and the historic falls structure.

Continue on the path past the TISCO complex. You will cross the refurbished truss bridge and proceed toward the ruins of Union Forge, the Solitude House and Solitude falls.

You might wish to plan ahead and leave a canoe at the boat dock so that you can take a respite from walking and canoe around Lake Solitude. You might just get a glimpse of a bald eagle. Even if you're not canoeing, you will find benches to sit and enjoy the lake view.

Head back to the trail. This is a little tricky involving a short walk on River Road. You will pick up the Nassau Trail and head up the hill. Chances are you will find the climb a bit challenging. You will make your way to Borough-owned open space at Springside Farm. Depending on the time of year, you may find this site mostly overgrown with tall grass. The buildings are not safe, so please do not enter.

For the return trip, you can reverse the route or walk out Countryside Lane to East Main Street and head back to town.

Do plan to allow at least 2 – 3 hours to appreciate this trail. If you're short on time or looking for an easier walk, you can end at Solitude House. In fact, there is adequate parking next to Solitude House, so you may want to park there on another day to make the trek up the Nassau Trail to Springside Farm.

This is a history lesson and family outing all in one probably best suited to children ages 8 and up.

Fishing is permitted at Lake Solitude with the proper New Jersey Fishing license.

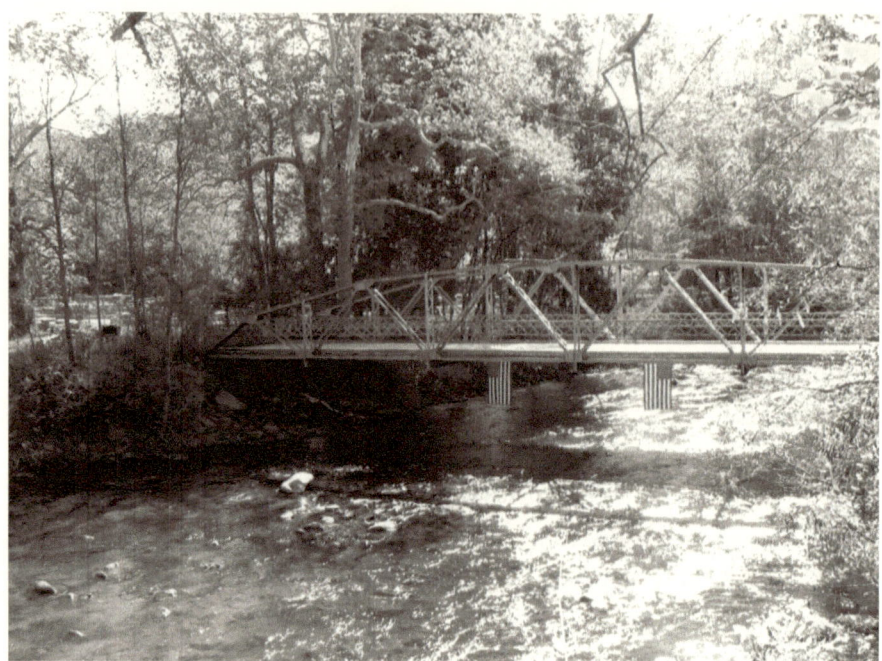

Jim Graham

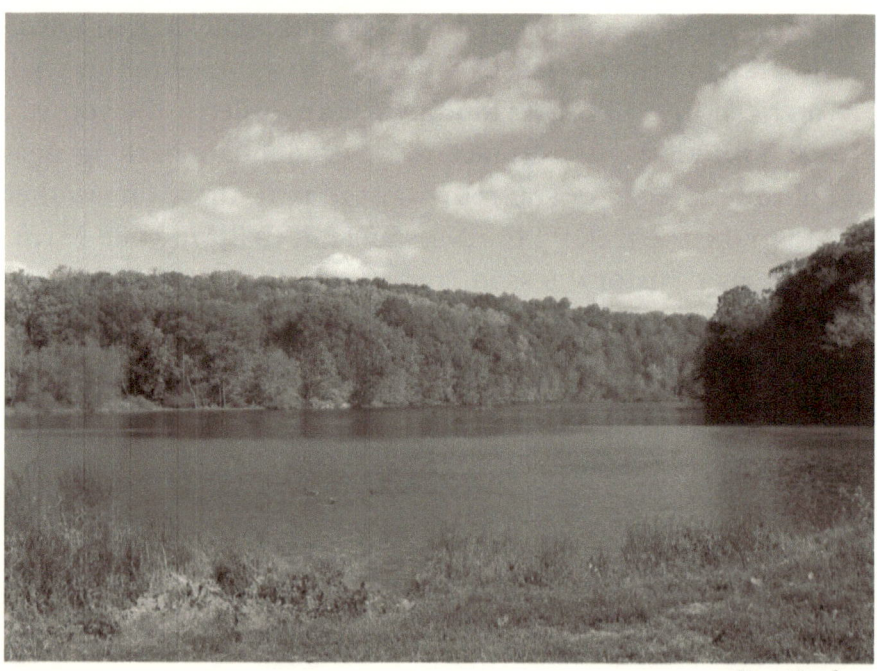

Jim Graham

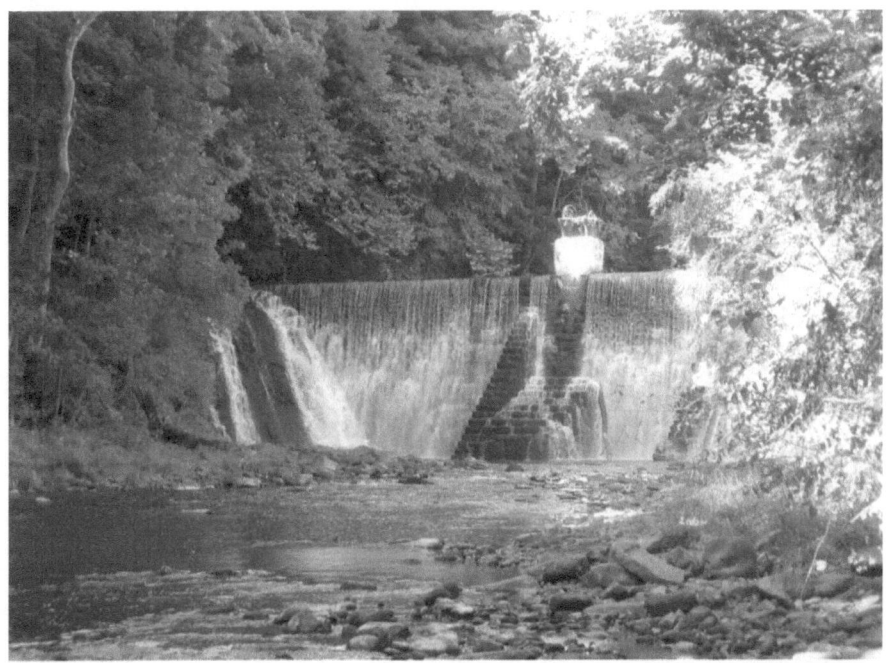

Jim Graham

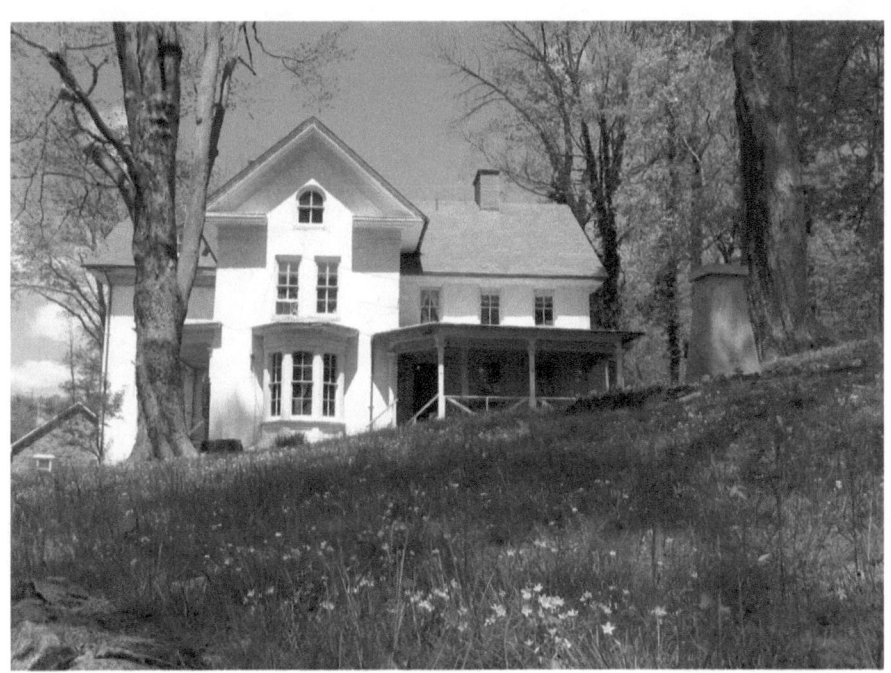

Mike Gronsky, Jr.

Alice Oldford

CHAPTER 5
UNION FURNACE PRESERVE

Government is instituted for the common good; for the protection, safety, prosperity, and happiness of the people; and not for profit, honor, or private interest of any one man, family, or class of men; therefore, the people alone have an incontestable, unalienable, and indefeasible right to institute government; and to reform, alter, or totally change the same, when their protection, safety, prosperity, and happiness require it.
John Adams, Thoughts on Government, 1776

Difficulty: Moderate to Difficult
Distance: 3 miles +
Location: Union Township
Sun/Shade: Mostly shade
Highlights: Views, reservoir
Restrooms: Not at this location, but available at Spruce Run Recreation Area
Parking: Paved
Hunting: Yes

Directions:

> From Rt. 31North or South, take VanSyckel's Road. Park in a designated spot on the left, opposite Union Furnace Preserve. If you like, park a second car at Spruce Run Recreation Area.

Cross the street from the parking area and enter the Union Furnace Preserve, which is well marked. The Preserve consists of 97 acres, and it is named for the ironworks which operated here from 1742-1781. The original entrepreneurs, William Allen and Robert Turner, were Loyalists who fled during the Revolutionary War. Robert Taylor, founder of Taylor Wharton Foundry in High Bridge, took over this ironworks. The actual furnace is under Spruce Run Reservoir.

Follow the trail up the embankment of an old mill race. This does get steep. Do keep the teal blazes in sight. You will come out on a cul-de-sac road called Serpentine Drive, and chances are you will enjoy the cool walk down the hill.

At Van Syckel's Road, turn left, then right into a parking area. You can stop here or add the Spruce Run Highlands Connector loop. If you decide to go on, you need to look carefully for the blazes. This is part of the Highlands Connector Trail, which is the subject of a loop hike described in "Spruce Run – Highlands Trail"

This is a nice, diverse hike – a bit strenuous as you hike up the embankment at Union Furnace Preserve. Then you finish with an easy walk along the reservoir. Whether you hike this half of the hike or merge this with the Spruce Run Connector, it is enjoyable and you will feel you have exercised after negotiating the embankment.

To control the deer population, hunting is permitted in the park with a special hunting license issued by the County Parks Department in addition to a New Jersey Division of

Fish and Wildlife license. Five permits are issued for the 97 huntable acres. Hunting is not permitted on Sundays. For complete details, please see the Hunterdon County Department of Parks and Recreation website, www.co.hunterdon.nj.us.

Alice Oldford

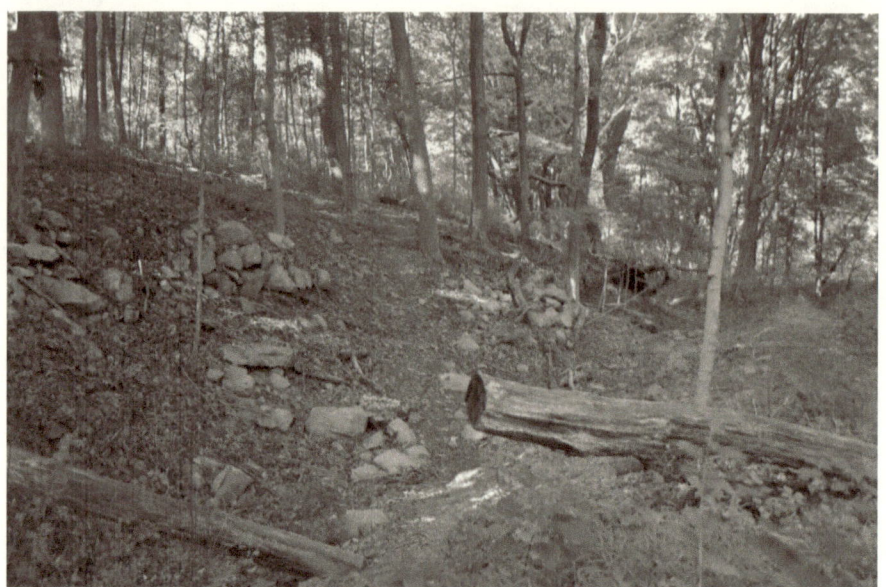

Laura Gooley-Trout

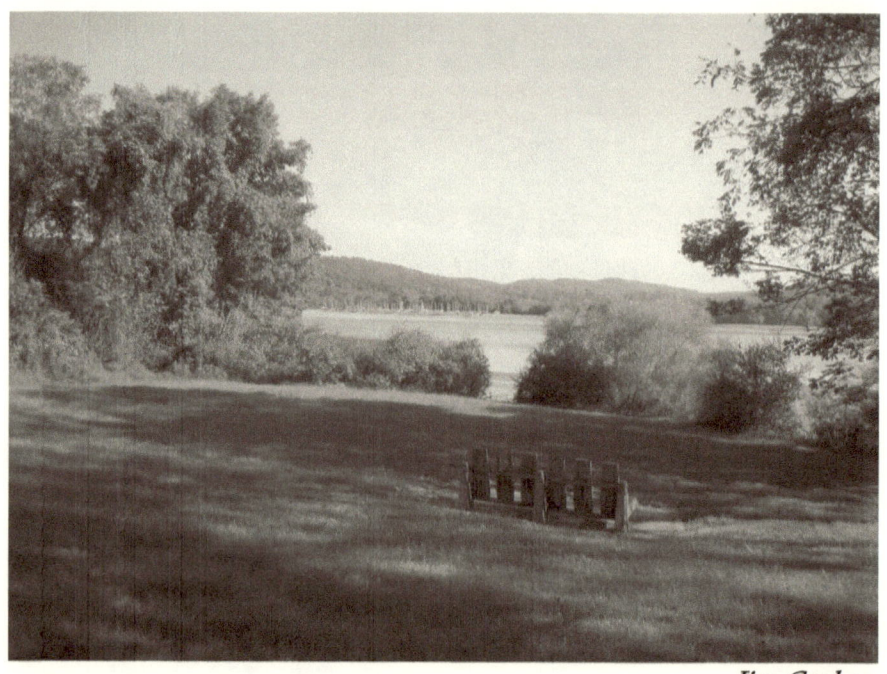

Jim Graham

CHAPTER 6
SPRUCE RUN – HIGHLANDS TRAIL

A lake is the landscape's most beautiful and expressive feature. It is Earth's eye; looking into which the beholder measures the depth of his own nature.
Henry David Thoreau

Difficulty: Moderate
Distance: 1.5–3 miles
Location: Clinton Township
Sun/Shade: Part sun/part shade
Highlights: Water, bird watching
Restrooms: Yes
Parking: Paved and gravel
Hunting: Yes
Directions:

> From Rt. 31North or South, take VanSyckel's Road to Spruce Run entrance

Spruce Run Recreation Area consists of 1290 acres with 15 miles of shoreline. It is the third largest reservoir in NJ after Round Valley and Wanaque Reservoirs. The earthen dam was completed in 1965.

Under the reservoir lie Lenape artifacts. Of additional historic significance, Union Iron Works, predecessor to

Taylor Wharton Iron and Steel Company of High Bridge was originally sited at Spruce Run until the Revolutionary Army dismantled the furnace. There is a marker for the site.

Although Spruce Run does not offer a trail system as part of its facility, it does host some portions of the Highlands Trail.

A loop hike is possible with a little ingenuity. This can be a pleasant, easy segment suitable for family. I suggest the two-car approach if possible. Leave one car in the Spruce Run Recreation lot and the other car in an unmarked, small lot (second one on the left when you enter VanSyckel's Road from Rt. 31).

You've parked the cars, and you are wondering whether it is worth the trouble. I predict you will be glad you did. Start from the unmarked lot. As you approach the water, look carefully and you will see the teal blaze. This is a lovely, easy single-track walk through meadows, a pine plantation and autumn olive thickets with views of the reservoir all along the way.

You will emerge near the group picnic area. Turn left when you reach the road and you will reach the Spruce Run parking area.

This is a 1.5 mile walk, and you can add another 1.5 miles by walking along the beach area toward the campsites. When you get to the boat rental area, loop back toward the parking area. If you've opted not to bring the second car, just head for the boat launch and make your way back to VanSyckel's Road for the walk back to the car.

This is especially nice to do off season – no cars, no entrance fee, few people. There are rest rooms in the Recreation area. Picnicking and/or playing on the beach are great options.

You can make this more challenging by connecting with the Union Furnace section, which is covered in Chapter 5.

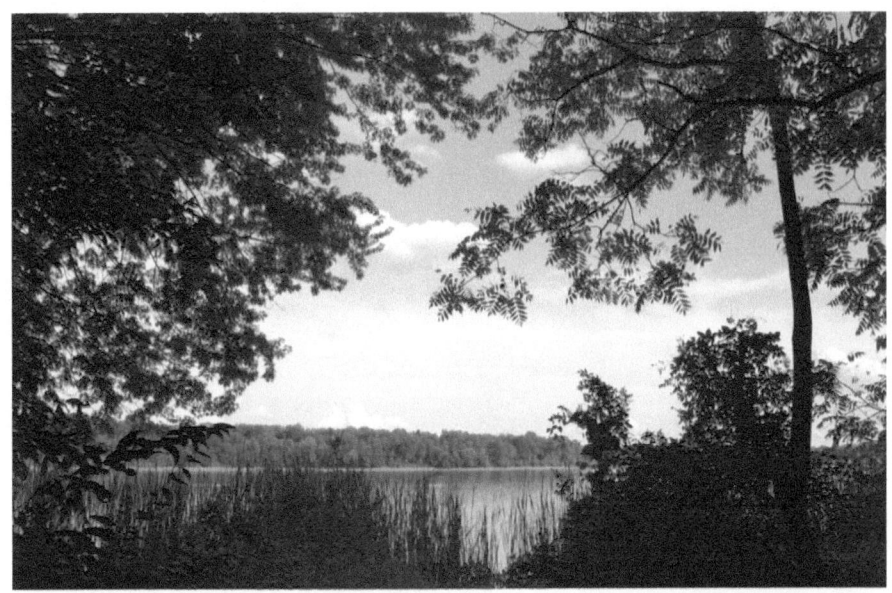

Laura Gooley-Trout

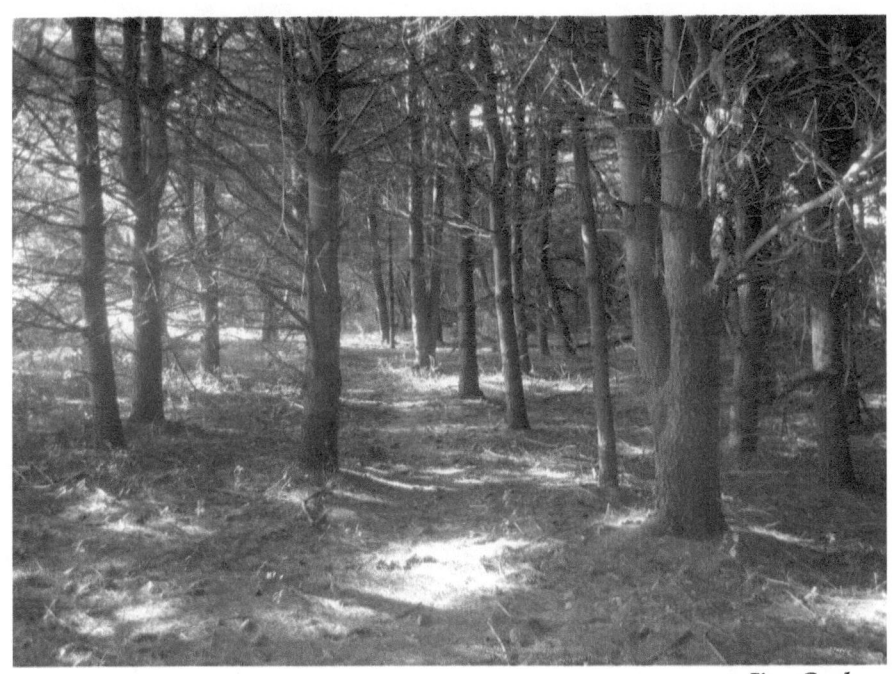

Jim Graham

Alice Oldford

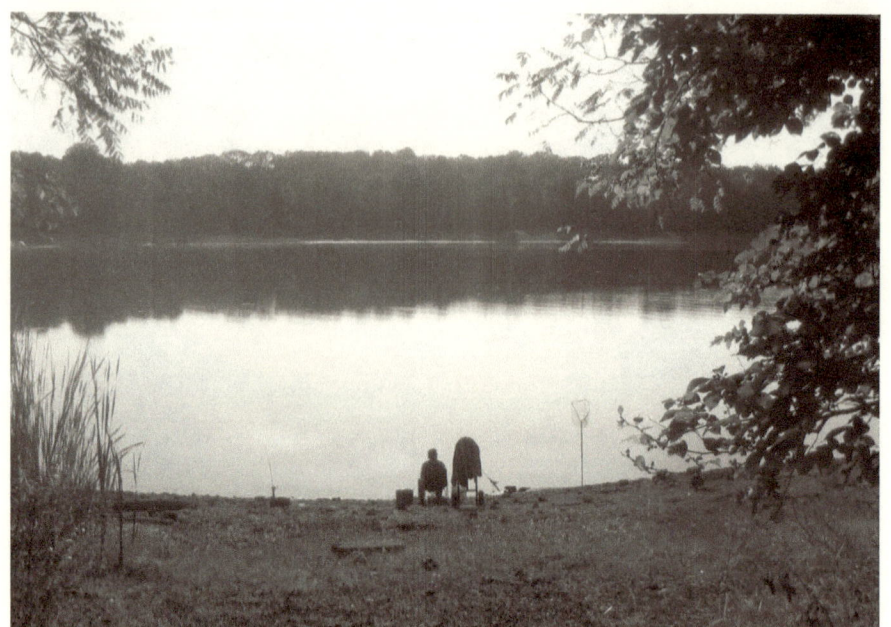

Jim Graham

CHAPTER 7
TOWER HILL RESERVE

Never doubt that a small group of thoughtful, committed citizens can change the world; indeed, it's the only thing that ever has.
Margaret Mead

Difficulty: Easy
Distance: Approximately 1 mile + connection
Location: Bethlehem Township
Sun/Shade: Mostly sun
Highlights: meadows, birds
Restrooms: no
Parking: yes, grass
Hunting: yes
Directions:

> From Clinton take Route I-78 west to exit 12. At the stop sign, turn left on Rt. 173 and then a quick right on Rt. 635. Proceed to the village of Norton and turn left on Norton Church Road. After a short distance, turn right onto Mountain View Road. Parking will be on the left.

A former farm, Tower Hill today comprises 216 acres of meadows, forested slopes and wetlands. You may want to combine this expedition with an outing to Jugtown Mountain Preserve found in my first book and included here for your convenience.

The County mapped hiking trail consists of approximately 1 mile around meadows. Long pants and hiking shoes are recommended.

Where it really gets interesting is connection on Mine Road to Highlands Trails. Follow the teal blazes. What appeared initially to be easy hiking quickly changes to moderate through the woods and over rocks. In one direction you access Jugtown Mountain Preserve where you continue to follow teal blazes across Rt. 173 to Tunnel Road.

In the other direction you can find your way to Spruce Run Recreation area approximately 8 miles.

I don't have a cool loop to suggest for this one, but you will find walking through the woods and along Mine Road to be pleasant. In the end you choose how long you want to spend exploring.

To control the deer population, hunting is allowed in the Park with a special hunting license issued by the County Park System in addition to the NJ Division of Fish and Wildlife license. There is NO hunting on Sundays. For complete details, please see the Hunterdon County Park System website, www.co.hunterdon.nj.us.

CHAPTER 8
JUGTOWN MOUNTAIN NATURE PRESERVE

Focus on remedies, not faults.
Jack Nicklaus

Difficulty: Moderate
Distance: 1.5 miles +
Location: Bethlehem Township
Highlights: Rocks, mining history, views
Restrooms: No
Parking: Dirt
Hunting: Yes
Directions from Rt. 78:

> Take Route 78 West to Exit 11. Proceed on Route 173
> west for about 2 miles. Turn right onto Mine Road.
> The entrance to the park is on the left just beyond
> the Bethlehem Township Building.

It is shady and cool, and the hiking is moderate at the
Jugtown Mountain Nature Preserve. You can hike the entire
trail in 1 hour. Hiking boots and long pants are
recommended.

Although we do not recommend this trail for young
children, we think it could be interesting to somewhat older

children, say 8 and up because of the interesting rocks, critters and perhaps the history. In some areas, depending on the time of year, there are locations where you can overlook the Musconetcong Watershed.

Wildlife habitat is abundant. See spotted salamanders and wood frogs that inhabit numerous vernal pools. The stonewalls and rock fields provide shelter to snakes and rodents.

Although its name identifies with moonshiners, who hid their jugs on rock ledges to avoid the authorities during prohibition, the history of the 153 acre preserve is in mining. The Swayze mine, which was located in the Preserve, was one of the top three producers of magnetic ore. At its peak, it produced 10,000 tons of ore annually before closing in 1889. You can still see remnants of mining activities including rock pits and ore dumps.

To control the deer population, hunting is allowed in the Park with a special hunting license issued by the County Park System in addition to the NJ Division of Fish and Wildlife license. There are 211 huntable acres, and 8 permits are issued. There is NO hunting on Sundays. For complete details, please see the Hunterdon County Park System website, www.co.hunterdon.nj.us.

CHAPTER 9
MUSCONETCONG GORGE PRESERVE

Don't judge each day by the harvest you reap, but by the seeds you plant.
Robert Louis Stevenson

Difficulty: Moderate to Challenging
Distance: 3 miles +
Location: Holland Township
Sun/shade: Mostly shade
Highlights: Waterfalls
Restrooms: No
Parking: Gravel on the side of the road
Hunting: Yes
Directions:

> West on I-78 to exit 7, pick up Rt. 173W approximately 1.3 miles to left on Rt. 639 approximately 4 miles. At the stop sign, bear left on Rt. 519, then turn left and cross the Musconetcong River staying on Rt. 519. Take next left on Dennis Road, a gravel road approximately .2 miles. Parking pull-off on the left.

The Musconetcong Gorge property consists of 425 acres originally owned by the paper mill, which is still in operation today.

This is a nice, shady hike in summer although the leaves preclude views of the River.

The waterfalls and other sources of water contribute to the cool feeling. If you've hiked at Point Mountain, chances are you will feel right at home at Musconetcong Gorge.

Long pants, hiking shoes and bug spray are strongly recommended for summertime walking. I believe it's too strenuous to be fun for the under 6 or 7 age group.

Although the trails are well marked, by all means take along a map to help you keep your bearings. We started out by bearing right toward the Ridge Trail. We tend to like doing the steepest sections first. We took the Ridge Trail with an aside to the waterfall, then on to the Switchback Trail. Just when you're feeling the need for a little break, you encounter the Railroad Trail, which is flat and easy. Then follow the signs for the Gasline Trail and Nature Trail, which revert to moderate, back to the parking area.

The oak-hickory forest provides comfortable habitat for deer and squirrels as well as black bears. The ravine and water are home to reptiles and amphibians. Watch for birds and raptors as well.

Although, this does not represent significant mileage, I predict you will feel you have had a good hike.

This is also a location of a portion of the Highlands Trail developed as a cooperative effort of the New Jersey/New York Trail Conference to create connections for trails between Hunterdon and Passaic Counties. As a connector trail, this continues and does not really lend itself to a loop.

To control the deer population, hunting is allowed in the Park with a special hunting license issued by the County Park System in addition to the NJ Division of Fish and

Wildlife license. There are 487 huntable acres in Holland and Bethlehem Townships, and 25 permits are issued. There is NO hunting on Sundays. For complete details, please see the Hunterdon County Park System website, www.co.hunterdon.nj.us.

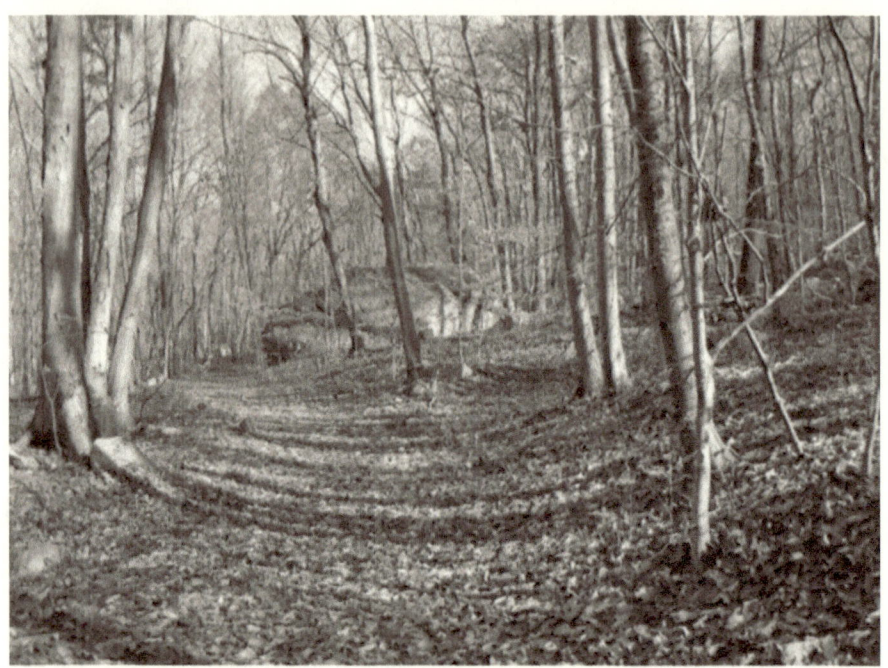

Jim Graham

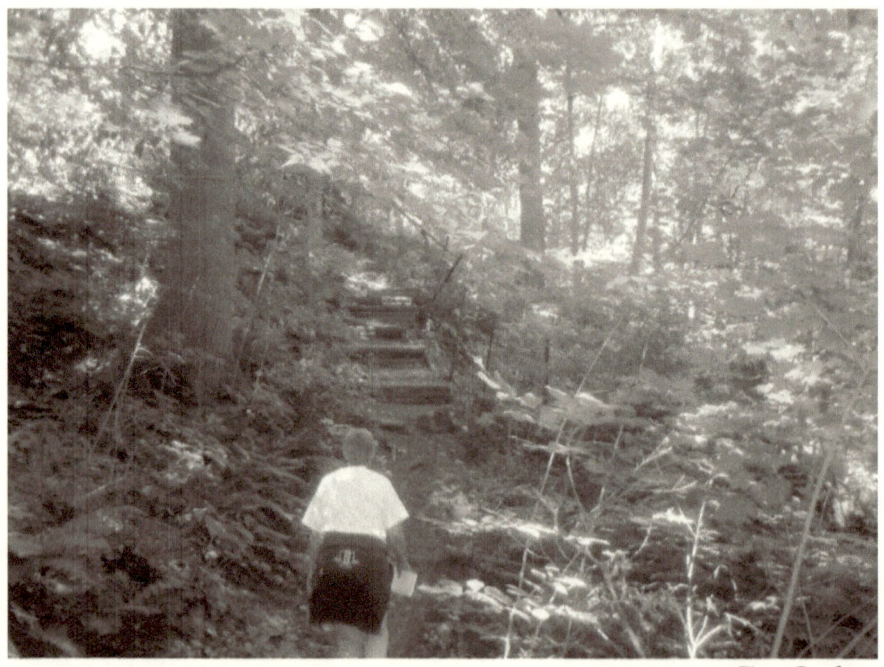

Jim Graham

CHAPTER 10
MINE BROOK PARK +
BERNADETTE MORALES NATURE PRESERVE
+ UPLANDS RESERVE

There is more to life than increasing its speed.
Mahatma Gandhi

Difficulty: Easy to Moderate
Distance: 3 miles
Location: Flemington Borough
Sun/Shade: Part sun/part shade
Highlights: Forest, wildlife, birding, creek views, playground equipment, pesticide free environment
Restrooms: Portajohn
Parking: Paved
Hunting: Yes – Uplands Reserve
Fishing: No
Directions:

> Rt. 12 to Old Croton Road to paved parking. Or Capner Street to paved parking.

What a terrific cooperative effort between Flemington-Raritan Parks and Recreation and Hunterdon County Parks Department. This parkland is part of a 400-acre greenway, including the Dvoor Farm, in the Flemington area. An added bonus is that Mine Brook and Morales are both part of pesticide free land.

There is something for everyone here in one place. There is plenty of paved parking at Mine Brook Park. If there are children who are looking to play ball, there is a playing field right there. Perhaps the age appropriate playground equipment is of interest to the younger set. In addition, there is a gravel fitness path that encircles the playing field. Generally, this path works for a stroller, but there are some spots that are a little deep. Consider yourselves warned. There are picnic tables and a pavilion in case you have a group needing some shelter from the sun or a sudden rain shower.

A nice walk starts at the parking lot and follows the path to the right around the ball field. Once you've made the circuit around the field, turn right and cross the bridge over the Mine Brook. This is also a great spot for kids to get close to the water and skip rocks or look for tadpoles.

Continue on up the hill until you reach the road. Don't be disappointed. The road walk is short. Turn left on the road, which is Shields Road and then left again at the next intersection of Capner Street. Follow Capner a short distance down the hill and cross the road to the Bernadette Morales nature trails. You can avoid the road altogether if you like by not crossing the bridge in the first place and following the gravel path to the Capner Street parking area.

The Morales nature trails are wide and well-marked with wooden posts. The footing consists of wood chips. Enjoy any of the options.

If you are inclined to continue to walk, follow the Meditation Trail, which is dirt with roots protruding. This leads to the County Uplands Reserve. Part of this is a paved farm road. After you've circuited the Uplands Reserve, you will make your way back to the Morales nature trails and back to the parking lot.

The route from Mine Brook Park, over the bridge, down Capner into Morales, then the Uplands and back through Morales is approximately 1 hour of easy to moderate hiking. It's probably not a great choice for the very young, but it is a nice option for 8 – 12 year olds as well as adults. Sturdy shoes are recommended.

To control the deer population, hunting is permitted in the Uplands Reserve with a special hunting license issued by the County Park System in addition to the NJ Division of Fish and Wildlife license. There is NO hunting on Sundays. For complete details, please see the Hunterdon County Park System website, www.co.hunterdon.nj.us.

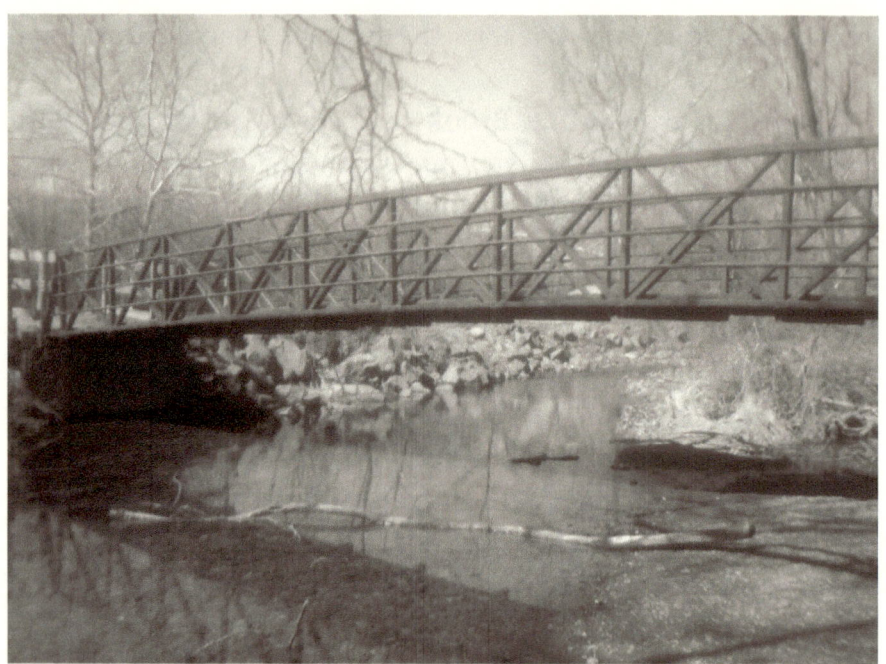

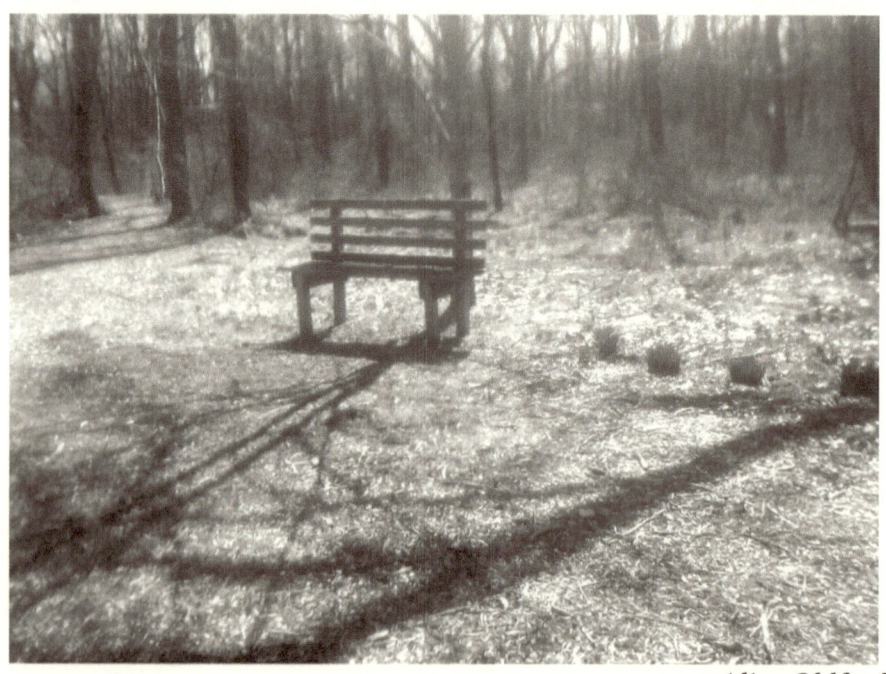

CHAPTER 11
DELAWARE & RARITAN CANAL STATE PARK
FEEDER CANAL

Be the change you want to see in the world.
Gandhi

Difficulty: Easy
Distance: Up to 31 miles one way
Location: Frenchtown Borough into Pennsylvania
Sun/Shade: Part Sun/Part Shade
Highlights: river views, historic landmarks
Restrooms: porta johns located sporadically
Parking: yes, paved
Hunting: limited
Directions:

> From Flemington take Route 12 west to
> Frenchtown. Parking area is on Bridge Street just
> before the bridge.

Oh the possibilities!

The canal and its structures were entered on the National Register of Historic Places in 1973, and the Delaware and Raritan Canal State Park became part of the

National Recreation Trail System in 1992.

The canal was constructed mostly by hand beginning in 1830 and completed in 1834 to transport cargo between Philadelphia and New York. There were two sections, totaling 70 miles, consisting of the Main Canal and Feeder Canal. In the beginning mule teams pulled the barges and canal boats – definitely slow going. By the end of the 19th century canal use was overtaken by the speed and power of railroads, and shipping was entirely discontinued in 1932. At that time the State of New Jersey took over the waterway and rehabilitated it to serve as a water supply system.

In 1974 over 60 miles of the canal and a narrow strip of land on both banks were made a state park.

One of my favorite walks/bike rides starts from Bridge Street in Frenchtown. Frenchtown is a destination in itself. Whatever interests you – books, antiques, restaurants, wine, eclectic gifts, even bicycle rentals – you will find in Frenchtown. I recommend you allow yourself some time after walking for browsing and partaking in some refreshment.

You're in charge of the distance. Head south. Unless you are very ambitious you probably will not find yourself in Pennsylvania, but do pick up a trail map and you may find you start from a different trail head for another expedition. This is an out and back walk, or it works very well for a point to point if you choose to use two cars.

The trail is wide, and the surface is mostly fine quarry process suitable for walking, biking, strollers. I don't think you need to worry so much about ticks as long as you stay on the trail, but you will probably be happy for some bug spray in summer, and I always recommend at least sneakers for footwear.

On another day tubing the Delaware is great fun with Delaware River Tubing http://www.delawarerivertubing.com

launching at the Kingwood Fishing Access where there is a porta john.

I love visiting Prallsville Mills, a 19th century mill complex operated by the Delaware River Mill Society. Keep an eye out at www.drms-stockton.org for activities conducted at Prallsville Mills.

Bull's Island Recreation area offers a day use area, campgrounds and the Bull's Island Natural area. It's also a place to launch boats into the canal and the Delaware River. Cross a pedestrian bridge over the Delaware River into Pennsylvania. There is an informational building with restrooms.

What a choice for outings. Lambertville is also a good place to start or Washington Crossing State Park, which is a park for all seasons. Many people make an annual visit on Christmas Day for a re-enactment of Washington crossing the Delaware.

Enjoy your sojourn in the D & R Canal State Park.

Alice Oldford

CHAPTER 12
WHITE OAK TRAIL +
RAVEN ROCK-LOCKATONG CREEK TRAIL SYSTEM

The key to happiness is having dreams. The key to success is making dreams come true.
Anonymous

Difficulty: Easy to Moderate
Distance: 3 miles +
Location: Kingwood Township
Sun/Shade: Mostly shade
Highlights: Forest, wildlife, creek views
Restrooms: Yes at Bull's Island State Park
Parking: Paved
Hunting: Yes
Fishing: Yes
Directions:

> Follow Rt. 29 South past Frenchtown. Parking for Bull's Island is on the right.

First, kudos to Delaware Township for developing and clearly marking the White Oak Trail.

The history of this area dates to the Lenape of the Unami

Indians. By the early 1700s the property in the area supported a farming community known as Saxtonville. In 1834 the opening of the Delaware and Raritan canal allowed for transportation of people and goods to Trenton, a 23 mile trip. In 1854 the railroad had stops at Bull's Island and Stockton, and the area evolved from strictly farmland to include a quarry operation, a railroad station, waterway stop, 2 stores, 2 inns, a tavern, a covered bridge, a post office and 12 dwellings. The community acquired a new name, Raven Rock.

There are so many options to explore, and we would like to broaden your horizons from Bull's Island and the scenic canal path to the White Oak and connecting trails. You will need to use a little ingenuity to make a loop. Parking at Bull's Island is a good choice. Proceed from the parking area across Rt. 29 at Quarry Road and go south a short distance. You will see a sign for the White Oak Trail, and it is a well-marked path through the woods with points of interest marked along the way. This trail is probably most enjoyable when the weather has been dry, and it is certainly a scenic choice in the fall.

Hiking shoes are recommended. You will be going up. This is likely not a fun place for small children, but I suspect children over 6 will enjoy the diversity.

The trail is an out and back trail, but you could loop by proceeding south on Federal Twist Road to Quarry Road and back to the parking area. There is very little traffic on the roads, and they do provide an interesting walk.

When you reach the end of the .9 mile trail, you may wish to extend your walk. The connection to the Raven Rock-Lockatong Creek Trail System is easy to make. When you step out on Federal Twist Road, make a left on Raven Rock-Rosemont Road and proceed to a parking area on the left. From this point you can access Mimi's Trail, a one-mile trail through the Zega-Lockatong Preserve which meanders along the Lockatong Creek. This is a shady pleasant walk. Again, this trail does not loop. However, you could cross the brook, assuming the water is low enough and access the Raven Rock-Rosemont Road back to Federal Twist and Quarry Road.

If you're really feeling adventurous and you have the time, Mimi's Trail connects to the Wescott Preserve, which then connects the beginning.

A second car option is definitely a possibility, parking either at Raven Rock-Rosemont Road or Strimples Mill Road.

We did find the road portions of the routes enjoyable because there is little traffic, generous shade and interesting houses and barns along the way.

Just as a matter of reference, you are parking on State property, starting the White Oak Trail which was developed by Delaware Township, proceeding on Mimi's Trail developed by Hunterdon Land Trust Alliance and finishing in Wescott Preserve a Hunterdon County Park system trail and Ralph Peter's Trail which is jointly owned by Hunterdon County Parks Department and Hunterdon Land Trust Alliance. You will see that there are different markers for each of these trails.

To control the deer population, hunting is permitted in a designated area of the park separate from the Day Use Area with a license issued by the New Jersey Division of Fish and Wildlife. For complete details, please see the NJ Division of Fish and Wildlife site.

Fishing in the Lockatong Creek is allowed year round, and it is stocked spring and fall with brown, rainbow and brook trout. NJ Division of Fish and Wildlife rules apply.

CHAPTER 13
WHITTEMORE WILDLIFE SANCTUARY

Teaching children about the natural world should be seen as one of the most important events in their lives.
Thomas Berry

Difficulty: Easy to Moderate
Distance: 1 mile +
Location: Tewksbury Township
Sun/shade: Mostly shade
Highlights: Wildlife, wetlands
Restrooms: Yes
Parking: Gravel
Hunting: Yes
Directions:

> East on I-78 to exit 24 for Route 523N, to left on Rockaway Road, then first left. Follow a long driveway to designated parking.

This is for the kids!

The Sanctuary property was bequeathed to Tewksbury Township by Helen A. Whittemore, and the site is dedicated to environmental education. The Township maintains the property. A non-profit 501c(3) organization, The Friends of

Whittemore, T/A The Roving Nature Center offers environmental education programs to children of all ages. Do check out their website www.rovingnature.com for educational programs ongoing throughout the year. The home office is located on the grounds of the Whittemore Wildlife Sanctuary.

Eleven miles of hiking trails, primarily through the woods, are available. Be aware that there are wetland areas to cross, and there could be high grass, so do go with long pants and sturdy shoes. The trails are well marked, and there is a map so you can choose an easy stroll or something more challenging. Include the kids or take a hike while your kids enjoy an educational program.

Thanks to Tewksbury for maintenance and development and sharing this wonderful spot with the public.

Hunting on Township property is allowed by permit and is regulated by the Township Police in accordance with State Fish and Wildlife rules and regulations during hunting season. Hunting is prohibited on Sundays. Signs and schedules will be posted in the park during hunting season.

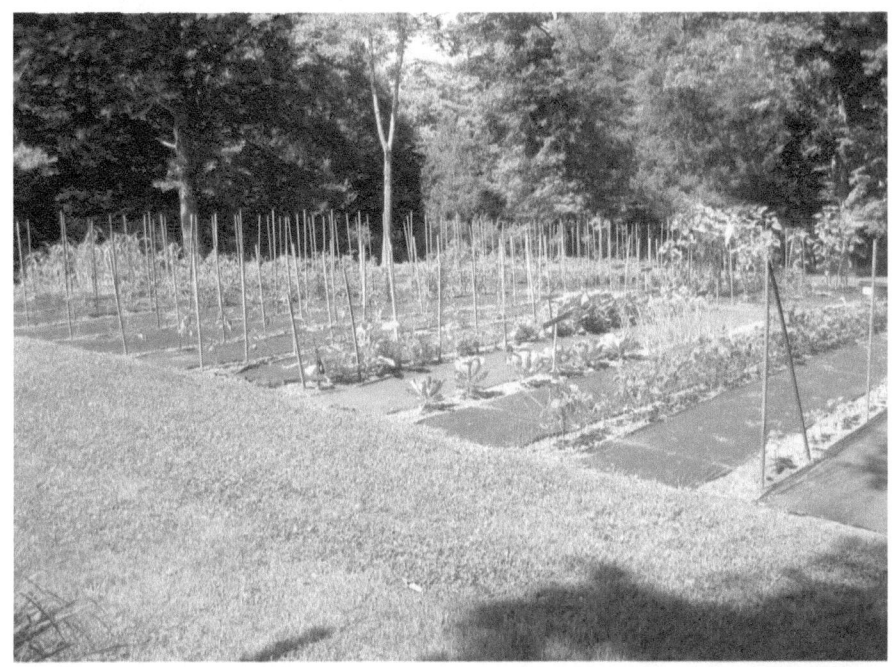

Jim Graham

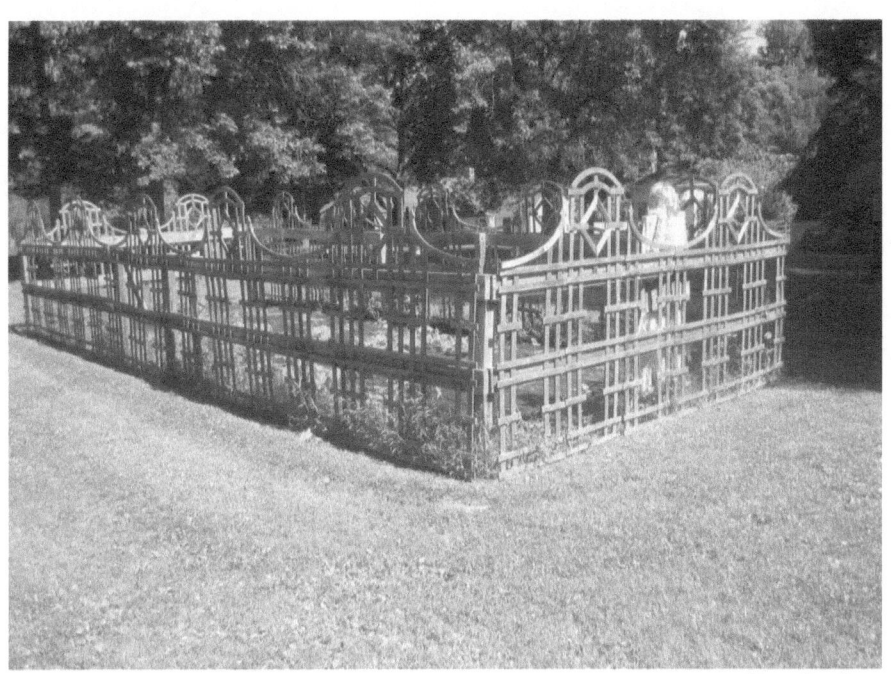

Jim Graham

Alice Oldford

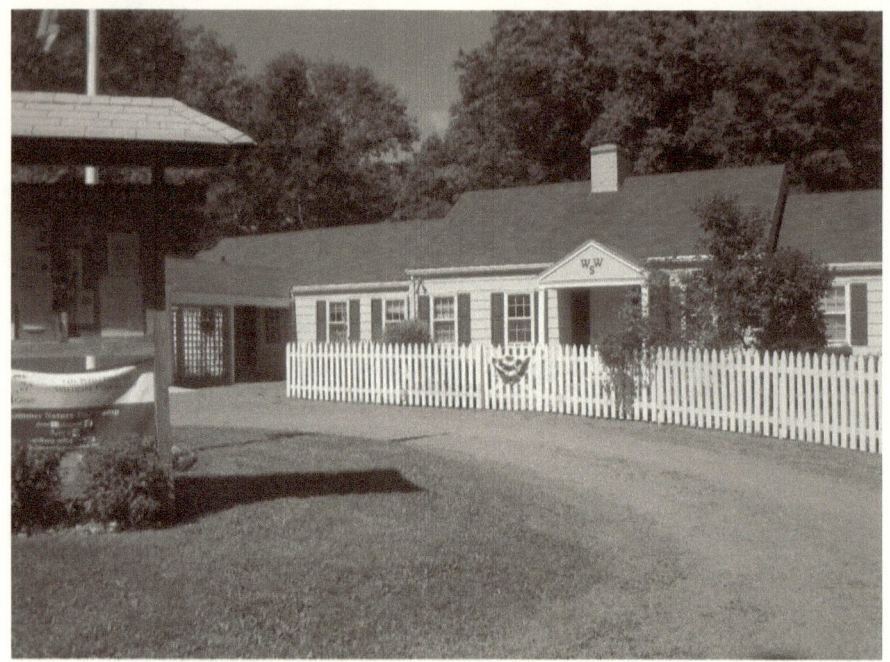

Jim Graham

WARREN COUNTY

CHAPTER 14
MERRILL CREEK RESERVOIR

Do not anticipate trouble or worry about what may never happen.
Keep in the sunlight.
Ben Franklin

Difficulty: Moderate
Distance: 5.5 miles
Location: Harmony Township, Warren County
Sun/shade: Sun and shade
Highlights: Views, eagles, visitor's center
Restrooms: Yes
Parking: Paved
Restrictions: No horses, bikes or motor vehicles
Hunting: Private Club – Merrill Creek Conservation &
Sportsmen Association
Boating: Electric Motors only
Directions:

Rt. 31 to Rt. 57W, 6.5 miles to right on Montana Road

Merrill Creek consists of 2000 acres with a 650 acre reservoir and 290 acre environmental preserve privately owned by Merrill Creek Owners Group who generously open this beautiful site to the public.

This is a lovely destination for your entire family. You are greeted by a wonderful Visitor's Center open daily from 8:30 a.m. to 4:30 p.m. and weekends 10:00 a.m. to 4:00 p.m. This is a treasure in itself suitable for a visit in any weather. Everyone in the family will find something of interest. Environmental education programs are available for pre-K through adults. Check with the office to find out what is being offered or arrange for a program for your group. (908) 454-1215 or admin@merrillcreek.com.

Perhaps it is a beautiful day, and you are looking for more of an outing. The hiking is great, offering so much diversity including woods, open fields some rocky single track trails. The topography is primarily level but there are some rolling areas. My favorite walk is a perimeter walk, which is 5.5 miles around the reservoir. You will need sturdy shoes, and I do recommend long pants. Of course, you will be happy to have along your water bottle, and a snack would be nice as well. Depending upon the weather, you may be well advised to have along some insect repellent. There are many spots to stop and enjoy a break.

There is a favorite viewing area for eagles and raptors. You can do this as part of your walk or make it a destination in itself. Eagle watchers report that Merrill Creek's resident bald eagles began their 13th nesting season in 2011.

Various short, marked trails, including a wheelchair accessible area, truly offer something for everyone in your family.

If fishing is of interest, the reservoir is the place to be with a boat. Shoreline fishing is prohibited. The reservoir is best known for its brown trout fishing. Rules for boating and fishing, the schedule of opening and closing hours, a depth map of the reservoir, and a list of regulations on fish catch are posted on the bulletin boards and also available at the Boat Ramp and the Visitors Center.

Whether you're looking for a couple of hours, half day or day long outing, you will not be disappointed.

Hunting is allowed for members of a private club and regulated by the rules of the New Jersey Division of Fish and Wildlife.

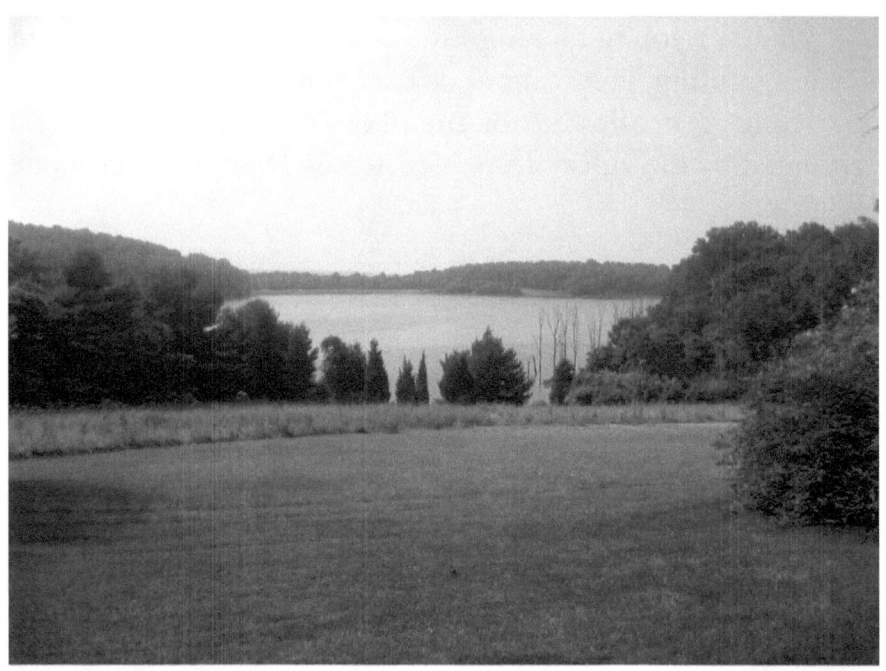

Jim Graham

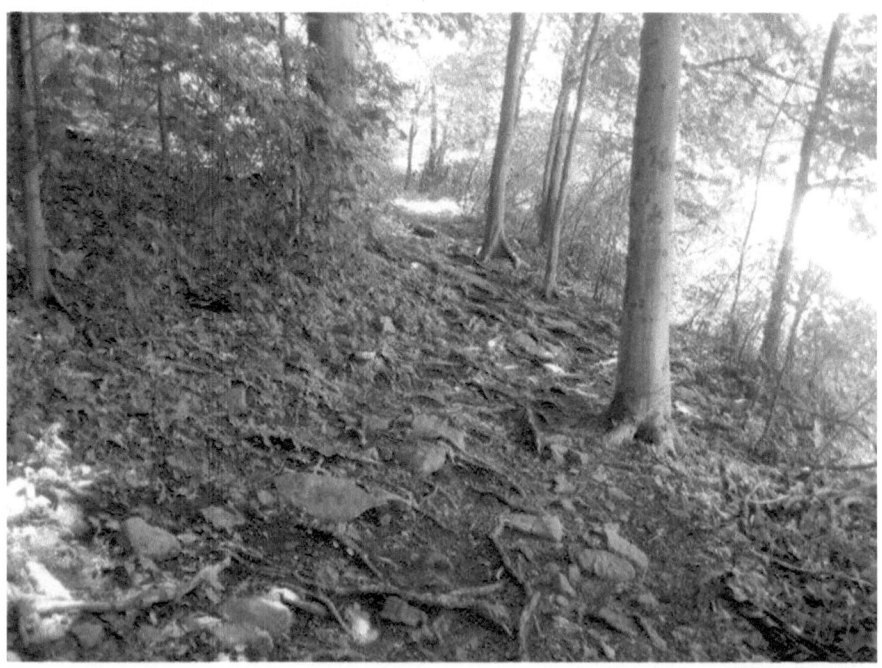

Jim Graham

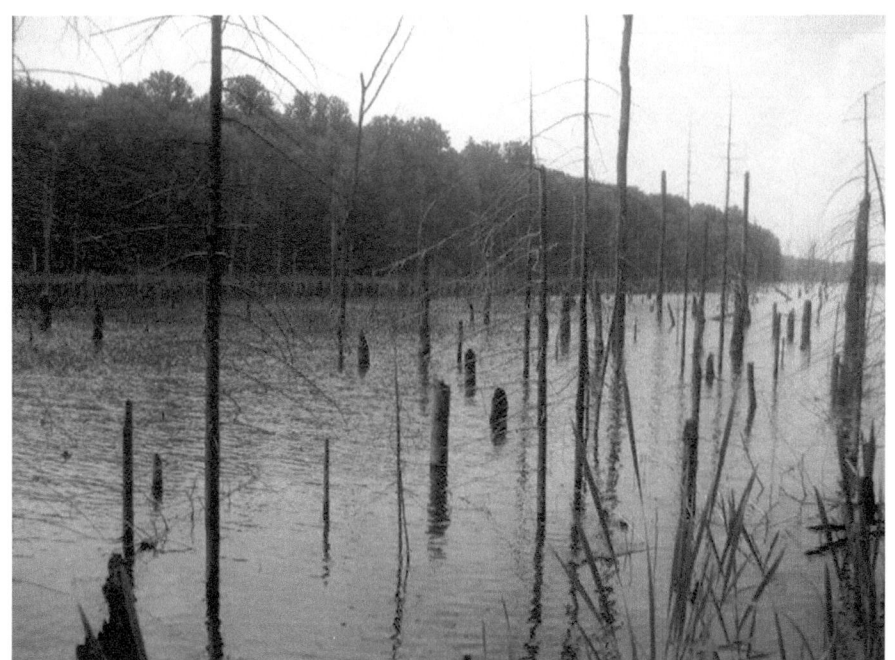

Jim Graham

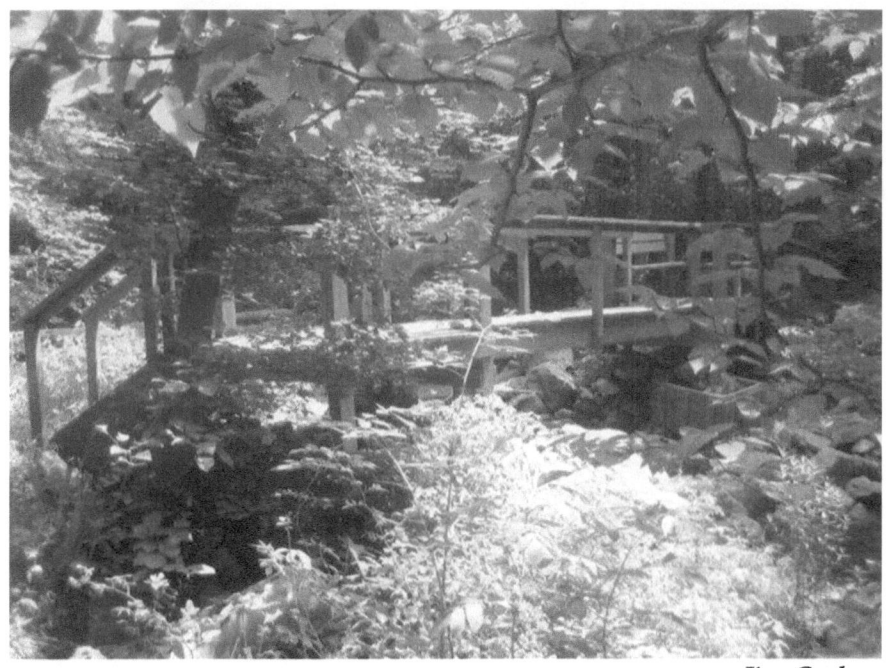

Jim Graham

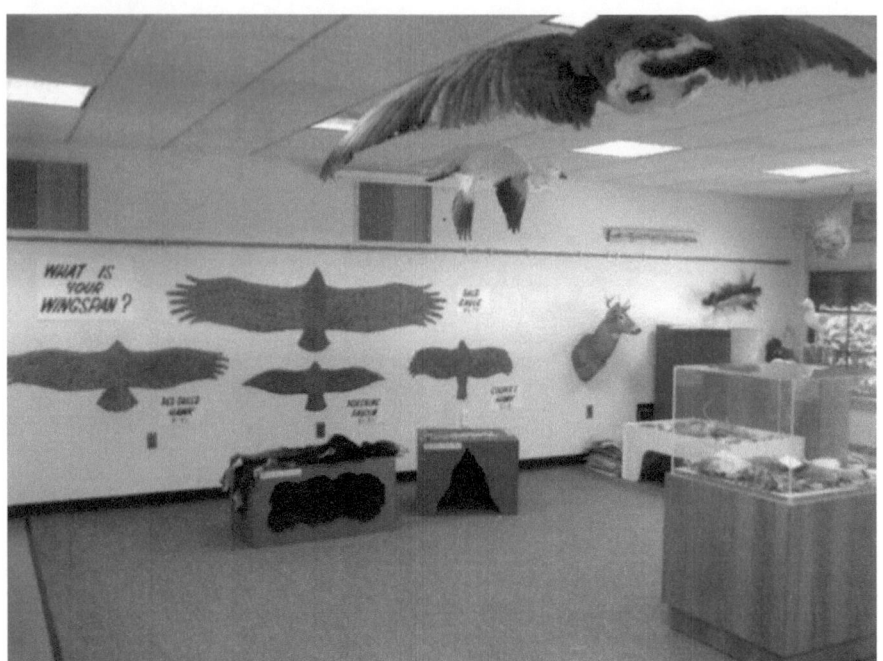

Jim Graham

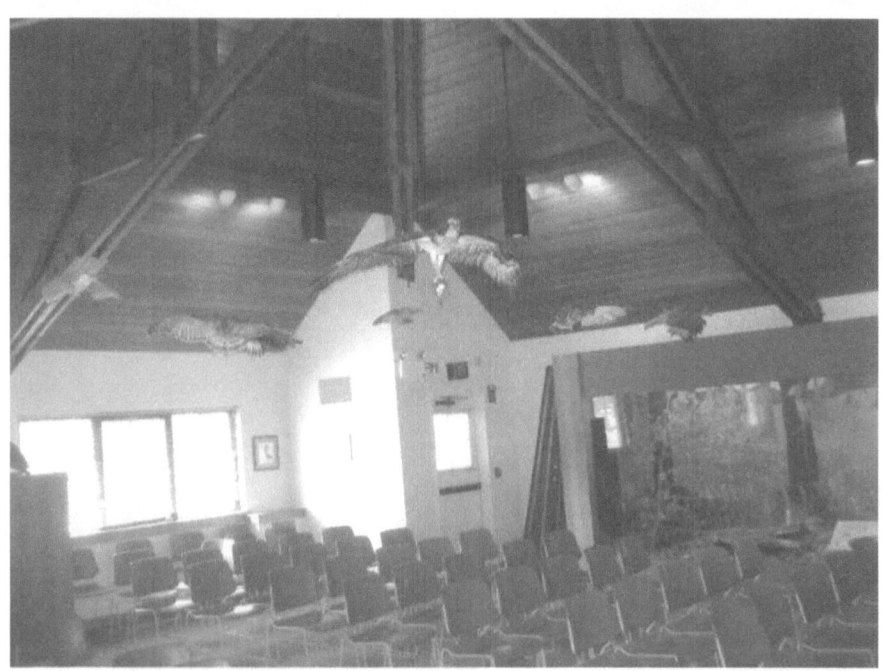

Jim Graham

MORRIS COUNTY

CHAPTER 15
HACKLEBARNEY STATE PARK
DAY USE AREA

Everybody needs beauty as well as bread, places to play in and pray in, where nature may heal and give strength to body and soul.
John Muir

Difficulty: Moderate
Distance: 3 miles +
Location: Long Valley and Chester Township
Sun/Shade: Mostly shade
Highlights: Forest, wildlife, river views
Restrooms: Yes
Parking: Paved
Hunting: Yes
Fishing: Yes
Directions:

>Follow Rt. 513 from Hunterdon County through Long Valley. It becomes Rt. 24 W. Turn right on State Park Road. Follow for 2 miles to park entrance on the left.

This beautiful, diverse State park now consists of 977 acres with hiking trails in the northern portion of the 465-

acre natural area. It originated in 1924 with 32 acres donated by Adolph Borie in memory of his mother and niece. Early development work was handled by the Board of Conservation and Economic Development. The High Bridge Civilian Conservation Corps Company 1268, who developed Voorhees State Park, continued work at Hacklebarney throughout the 1930's.

Restrooms are available close to the parking area as well as within the park. There are picnic tables and charcoal grills at various locations within the park. There is also a playground close to the parking area. The trails are well maintained.

Since there is so much to offer, you would be well served to have a plan before undertaking this Park. You could plan a family expedition, including some exploration and a picnic. Note you may select a remote picnic location which is a considerable hike from the parking area, so you may want to keep the picnic hamper light.

You may want to take a shady walk in the hemlock forests by the Black River. Steep ravines offer a great vantage point for river viewing and ideal exploration terrain for the younger set. You can certainly opt to do it all. The terrain is diverse depending on the distance you choose. For a nice overview, about 1 ½ hours, follow the red trail through the forest and be treated to a view of waterfalls and a walk along the Black River. Some of the walk near the river is rocky. Once you cross the Rinehart Brook, you can pick up the main trail and return to the parking area. If you are up for more adventure, there are options to continue.

Long pants and sturdy shoes are recommended, and insect spray would be handy in summer. This is a wonderful, peaceful walk in the fall.

To control the deer population, hunting is permitted in a designated area of the park separate from the Day Use Area with a licensed issued by the New Jersey Division of Fish and Wildlife. For complete details, please see the NJ Division of Fish and Wildlife site.

Fishing in the Black River is allowed year round, and it is stocked spring and fall with brown, rainbow and brook trout. NJ Division of Fish and Wildlife rules apply.

Hacklebarney, located within Morris County, is part of the State Park system.

I am impressed with Morris County Park Commission's ongoing development. Near Hacklebarney is Patriot's Path, which is an easy walk on well-marked trails. This park has yielded Indian artifacts, which are on display. Enjoy a visit to Cooper's Mill, which is open to the public during limited hours. Trail maps and visitation hours are available at http://www.morrisparks.net/parkslist.asp. Do check before you go to see what is new. Kudos for the Morris County Park Commission's commitment to development.

To control the deer population, hunting is permitted in designated areas of various Morris County parks between September and February. Morris County Park Commission typically prepares a hunting schedule in summer which is posted online. The list of parks allowing hunting changes annually, so do check before heading out. Signs are also posted in parking areas and at major trailheads.

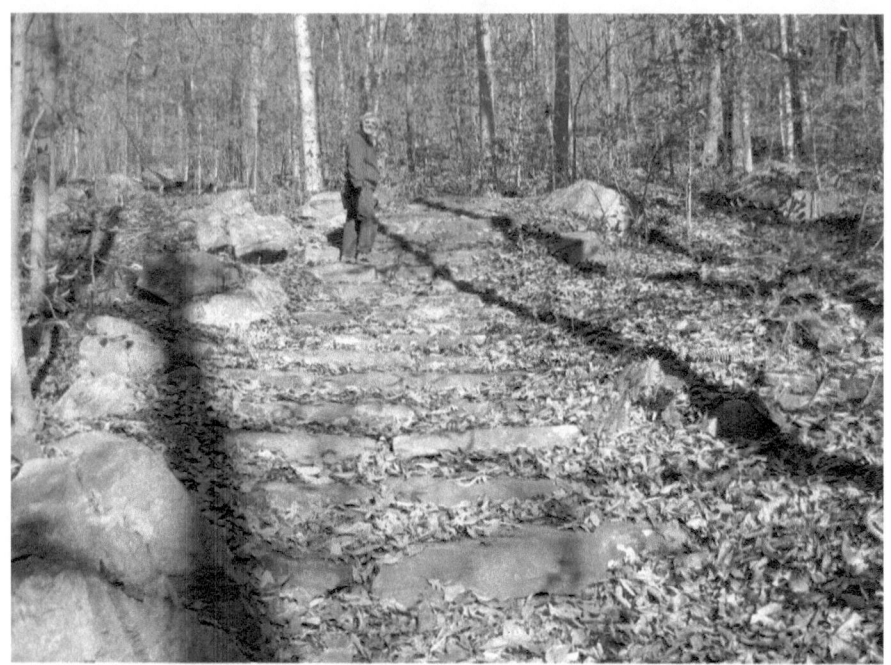

Jim Graham

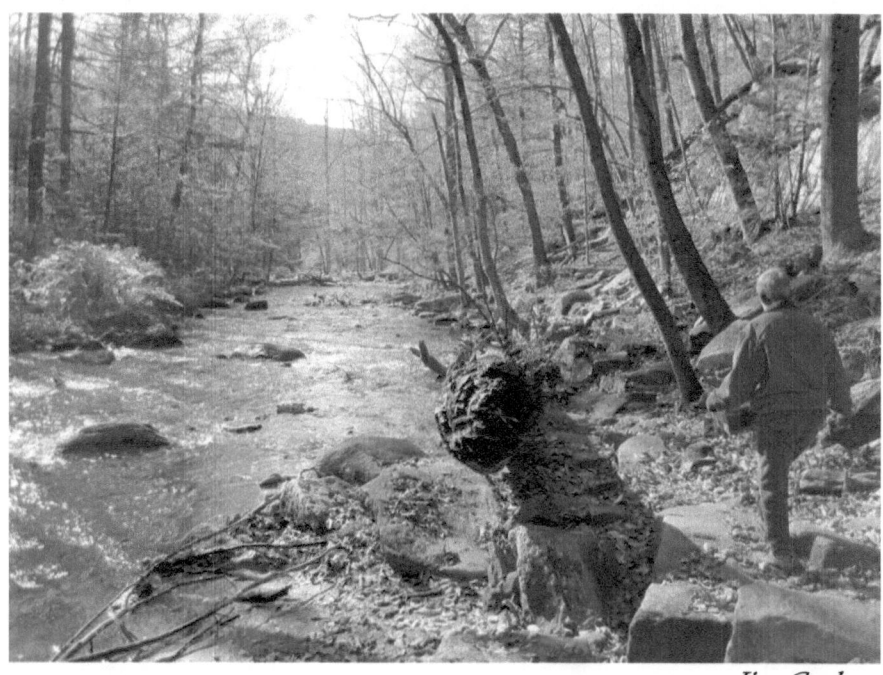

Jim Graham

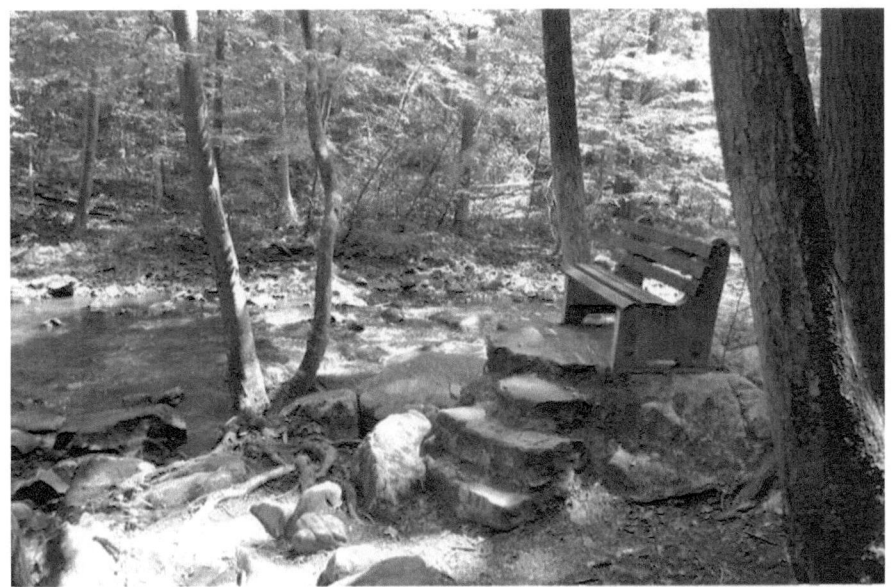

Laura Gooley-Trout

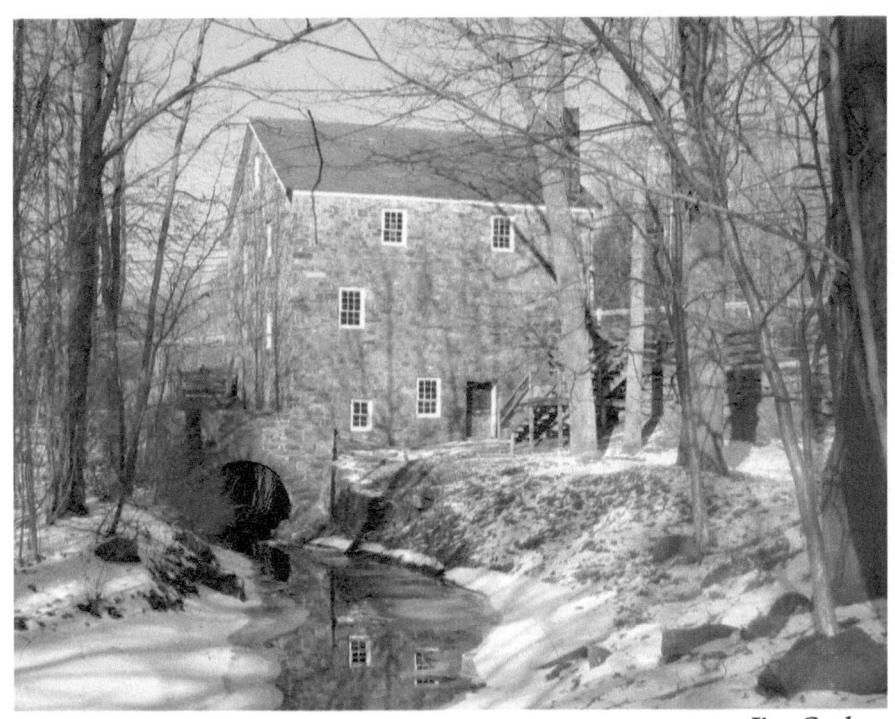

Jim Graham

Alice Oldford

HAPPY TRAILS TO YOU!

In every walk with nature one receives far more than he seeks.
John Muir

I hope this gets you outside smiling. It works for me, time after time, in all seasons.

This is just a sampling of our local trails. I am always thankful for those who have cared enough for nature and preservation to nurture the trail systems in New Jersey. I hope you will get hooked on the beauty and the exploration while embracing the seasonal and developmental changes.

Stewards of the various trails do a great job with limited budget keeping the trails user friendly.

Please do share your experiences on my website, http://www.get-there-from-here-books.com

Enjoy!